ALWAYS YOUNG

AF581538

JAMAL SIDDIQUI

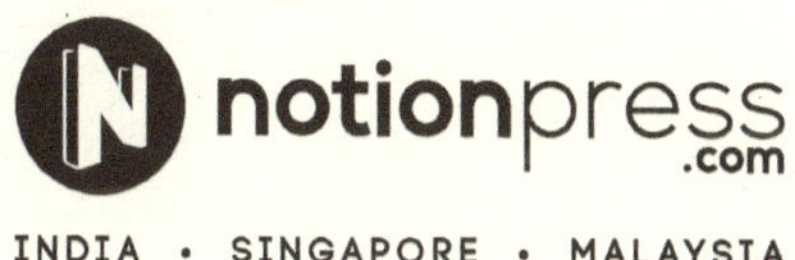

INDIA • SINGAPORE • MALAYSIA

Copyright © Jamal Siddiqui 2024
All Rights Reserved.

ISBN 979-8-89475-293-8

This book has been published with all efforts taken to make the material error-free after the consent of the author. However, the author and the publisher do not assume and hereby disclaim any liability to any party for any loss, damage, or disruption caused by errors or omissions, whether such errors or omissions result from negligence, accident, or any other cause.

While every effort has been made to avoid any mistake or omission, this publication is being sold on the condition and understanding that neither the author nor the publishers or printers would be liable in any manner to any person by reason of any mistake or omission in this publication or for any action taken or omitted to be taken or advice rendered or accepted on the basis of this work. For any defect in printing or binding the publishers will be liable only to replace the defective copy by another copy of this work then available.

Contents

About the Author

Jamal Siddiqui, born in Nirmal and educated in Hyderabad City, India, **has a rich cultural background**. He has traveled extensively abroad for over 25 years, but the United Kingdom and the Middle East remain his two favorite regions. He has cherished memories of India and considers Canada a delightful second home. **His academic journey is a testament to** his **intellectual prowess** and **dedication to learning**. He holds a Bachelor of Arts (BA) from Nizam College - Osmania University in Hyderabad and an (OM-MBA) from the USA. His decision to pursue higher education has honed his core competencies in writing. He furthered his academic journey with a Diploma in Journalism from London and a Bachelor of Laws (LL.B.) degree from London, England.

The Author has an impressive sports background, excelling as a cricketer and representing different levels of cricket championships. It's impressive to witness the passion for cricket **was evident from a young age, as they represented** the state **at** the under-19 years cricket, as well as their active involvement in the A Division league and their unwavering commitment to practice at the LB Stadium in Hyderabad, India. The commitment to physical fitness showcases a focus on performance and overall well-being.

Mr. Siddiqui's career path is a testament to his versatility and adaptability but also. He worked in the export management division of pharmaceutical multinational corporations. His role as an Author, Poet, & Journalist, and later in a law firm as a Legal Analyst Draftings & Pleadings, has further enriched his professional journey. His reflective writing on law and society has led to the publication of multiple articles in legal magazines and US-based e-newspaper. Mr. Siddiqui is the author of the books "Thoughts of Aesthetics," "Laughing Lawyer Clean Jokes," "Humour Station," and "Language of Heart Poetry," with another book set to be published at the end of 2024. Additionally, Mr. Siddiqui's English poetry has been included in many anthologies published in the US.

Introduction

Dear readers, I greet you with a pleasant and energetic welcome. The salutation represents the importance of well-being. I invite you to read this book to learn about physical fitness and its role in our lives.

Therefore, I urge you to start reading this book immediately. The knowledge and understanding you will gain from it are not just valuable, they are life-changing, and this choice will empower you to transform your life for the better.

The knowledge you acquire from this book is not just information but a valuable asset that will enhance your understanding of physical fitness and health, reassuring you that your investment in reading this book will benefit you and those around you.

Preface

To God alone be all the glory. This book was composed for individuals passionate about physical fitness and enjoying athletics. It **is a concise summary of** the benefits of exercise and the role of physical activities in today's world, with the required information about physical fitness, its importance, and its benefits. Before we delve into the content, I want to share my background. I come from a family with a rich athletic heritage. My father, M A Rasheed Siddiqui, was a soccer star at the university level. My late grandfather, M A Wahid Siddiqui, was a professional lawyer and had a deep passion for sports and was an exceptional swimmer. I, too, have a strong sports background, excelling as a cricketer and representing different levels of cricket championships. My passion for cricket was evident from a young age. I represented the State during the **under-19 years of cricket,** was actively involved in the A Division league, and had an unwavering commitment to practice at the LB Stadium in Hyderabad, India. Even today, I am dedicated to physical fitness, mainly through slow jogging. These personal experiences are the foundation of this book, and I hope they inspire and connect with you on your fitness journey.

This book is a culmination of my research and personal experiences, with all references provided on the bibliography page. It's a comprehensive guide to physical fitness, offering all general information and a message of health awareness. I want to clarify that this book is not my income source. I've published it and made it available on Amazon platform with the sole aim of reaching a global audience. The earnings from this book will be directed towards charitable causes, a testament to my belief in giving back to society. You can be reassured that this book provides a comprehensive and reliable source of information on physical fitness.

Despite advances in global development, many people are still unaware of their health and often ignore specific health issues, living in ignorance. This book is a guide for individuals affected by this lack of understanding, empowering them with the necessary information about the role of physical fitness in life. It aims to bridge the knowledge gap and empower readers with the knowledge they need to lead a healthy life.

The primary purpose of writing this book is to bridge the gap in understanding about physical fitness. In Asian countries, particularly India and Pakistan, there's a significant lack of awareness about physical fitness and its benefits. This book aims to fill that void, providing essential knowledge and insights that can help individuals lead healthier lives. By reading this book, you will be well-informed and enlightened about the importance of physical fitness, empowering you to make informed decisions about your health and well-being.

My respected father, Mr. M A Rasheed Siddiqui, admitted me into (L B Stadium) for cricket coaching and to practice cricket when I was just 14 years old; till today, I am doing physical fitness at least 3 days a week for 30 minutes daily.Further, the final reason for writing this book is that I have met many well-educated people with significant degrees, holding high positions and living luxurious lives. Still, they don't pay much attention to physical fitness. I have also seen many young girls who are unable to get married due to obesity because they don't spend any time on physical activities.

After reading this book, all readers, regardless of their age, think this book is for everyone, and it will help us appreciate the virtues and understand the importance of physical fitness.

Acknowledgements

I am thankful to Allah, who guided me on the right path and protected me from bad habits and gave me health awareness. I am grateful to my parents, who took good care of me throughout my childhood and provided me with the best upbringing; they have been a great source of encouragement. I especially value my father's advice on maintaining good health to live a good life, which has had a profound impact on me. I want to express my deep appreciation to my well-behaved children, Daughter Zeenath, for suggesting a good source of food and Son Nehaal, for their unwavering support and for pushing me to go for fitness regularly, as well as my son Nehaal, suggesting the front cover design.

Acknowledgments

Chapter One

What is Physical Fitness and Why is It Significant?

I started this topic with the two specific sayings of the Prophet Muhammed (PBUH) about Health; "Your body has a right over you", [1]- "There are two blessings that many people are deceived into losing: health and free time [2].

Physical fitness, a holistic approach to health, encompasses the overall well-being of an individual's body and mind. It entails the capacity to do everyday chores with enthusiasm and alertness, free from tiredness, and with enough energy to enjoy leisure-time activities and to handle unexpected events. It's not just about running a marathon or lifting heavy weights; it's about having a balance of strength, endurance, flexibility, and mental well-being. Achieving physical fitness requires consistent exercise, a healthy diet, enough sleep, and an optimistic outlook. Every person's path is unique and depends on their aspirations, skills, and way of living. Activities like running, strength training, yoga, or team sports can improve physical fitness. The benefits of physical fitness extend beyond just physical health; they also positively impact mental health by releasing endorphins like dopamine, which can improve mood and reduce stress. Cultivating an optimistic outlook is a key component of this holistic approach to health, enhancing the quality of life and promoting longevity.

Physical fitness, a holistic approach to health, encompasses the overall well-being of an individual's body and mind. It's about finding the capacity to do everyday chores with enthusiasm and alertness, free from tiredness, and with enough energy to enjoy leisure-time activities and to handle unexpected events. It's not just about running a marathon or lifting heavy weights; it's about balancing strength, endurance, flexibility, and mental well-being. Physical fitness requires consistent exercise, a healthy diet, enough sleep, and an optimistic outlook. Every person's path is unique and depends on their aspirations, skills, and way of living. Whether it's running, strength training, yoga, or team sports, the benefits of physical fitness extend beyond just physical health; they also positively impact mental health by releasing endorphins like dopamine, which can improve mood and reduce stress. Cultivating an optimistic outlook is a critical component of this holistic approach to health, enhancing the quality of life and promoting longevity.

It's a regrettable reality that such occurrences are widespread in Asian countries,specifically in my city, Hyderabad, India. Many individuals in Hyderabad struggle to find time for physical fitness. People in Hyderabad city do not spare 3 hours for physical fitness out of 1 week = 7 days, 168 hours a week. It's really disappointing how often people overlook the importance of their health. It's one of life's most valuable gifts; no money can restore it once it's lost. Surprisingly, most people, about 80 out of 100, either disregard this fact or simply don't prioritize it due to their busy schedules. However, please prioritize your health by dedicating three hours weekly to maintaining your well-being. Physical fitness offers many benefits, including a boost in energy levels and enhanced mental well-being. I encourage you to personally witness these advantages, feel inspired, and make a change in your life.

Please note: I am not a fitness specialist or trainer. However, I have gained knowledge in this area from my school and university and, most importantly, from my personal journey with fitness. This personal experience, which has shaped my understanding and belief in the importance of physical fitness, is what drives me to share this message with you.

In sharing this knowledge, I urge you to prioritize your health. My final recommendation to my readers is that a good diet and regular exercise make a man healthy and happy. A good diet is not just about what you eat, it's about what you are. It's about making informed choices that empower you to live your best life. Your health is invaluable, and I want you to know that I deeply care about your well-being.Physical exercise is not just a routine, it's a key to unlocking a healthier, happier you. It offers a myriad of benefits such as increased muscle strength, improved flexibility, enhanced stamina, and a healthier heart. It's a powerful tool for weight management and can even alleviate depression. So, lace up your shoes and let's embark on this journey to a better you.

Adopting a balanced diet and incorporating regular exercise is not just a religious duty but also a powerful tool for taking control of our health. It's a scientifically proven method for maintaining optimal health. In today's society, it is unfortunate that many individuals tend to neglect their health concerns, such as obesity, until they are faced with more severe ailments like type 2 diabetes. However, prioritizing physical fitness can significantly decrease the likelihood of health problems and assist with weight loss and management. This empowerment is a crucial aspect of our journey toward optimal health, and it's a journey that each of us, as individuals, are responsible for and engaged in. Let's delve into each benefit of physical fitness: Research has indicated that people who maintain a physically active lifestyle generally experience extended lifespans and improved overall well-being. Prioritizing physical fitness is vital for preventing chronic illnesses and improving general well-being.

For those who neglect their health by consuming excessive sugar, a poor diet, and indulging in junk food, it's time to take a serious look at the potential dangers to your health. Research shows that these factors not only impact you physically but also affect your mental well-being. Remember, physical exercise is a highly individualized journey, with unique benefits for each of us. The key to good health is finding the right exercise balance for your age and lifestyle and making it a daily habit. The duration and intensity of a physical workout can bring about various benefits, each unique to you. With its wide-ranging advantages, physical fitness can lead to a heightened sense of satisfaction, a more relaxed state of mind, and a refreshing feeling after each session. These unique benefits are what make physical fitness a holistic journey that offers numerous advantages to your body, encompassing mental, physical, and spiritual aspects. It helps you cultivate healthier habits like regular physical activity and proper eating while reducing the risk of type 2 diabetes and circulatory issues, giving you hope for a healthier future.

Participation in physical fitness at the age of 40:

A subtle reminder to individuals to prioritize their physical fitness as they approach the age of 40. This is because the body undergoes various changes as it ages, such as decreasing muscle mass, slowing metabolism, and increasing the risk of diseases like heart disease and diabetes. Regular exercise may help fight these changes and improve health. For instance, a study published in the Journal of the American Medical Association found that regular exercise can reduce the risk of heart disease by 30%. It can also help maintain muscle strength, flexibility, and bone density, essential for preventing injuries and maintaining independence at one age. Maintaining good health over forty has several benefits, including a lower risk of age-related chronic diseases and other conditions. Learn the extraordinary advantages of integrating consistent exercise into your daily routine. Begin your journey toward a healthier and joyful you by bidding farewell to obesity, diabetes, hypertension, and heart disease.

Moreover, by engaging in cardiovascular exercises like brisk walking, swimming, or cycling, strength training exercises such as weightlifting or bodyweight exercises, and flexibility exercises like yoga or stretching, individuals can enhance their quality of life, improve their longevity, and experience the joy and fulfillment of a healthy lifestyle. Regular exercise can mitigate the risk of age-related health issues, making you feel more motivated and inspired to take charge of your health. Reassure yourself that by prioritizing physical fitness after age 40, you are making a confident and beneficial decision for your health.

Walking is best

Engaging in regular walks can greatly enhance one's overall health and well-being. It's a straightforward yet efficient form of exercise that provides numerous advantages. As you walk, you activate different muscles in your body, gradually enhancing their strength. This can result in enhanced muscle strength and improved stamina. In addition, walking is an excellent form of cardiovascular exercise. Increasing your heart rate has numerous benefits, including enhancing heart health and promoting better circulation. Engaging in regular walking can contribute to maintaining a healthy weight and lowering the chances of developing chronic conditions such as diabetes and heart disease. One of the greatest advantages of walking is how easily accessible it is. It can be done in various locations and at any time, without requiring any specific equipment. It's a gentle exercise that can be enjoyed by individuals of varying fitness levels. In addition, walking can have a positive impact on mental well-being by helping to alleviate stress and anxiety. It's a wonderful way to refresh your thoughts and appreciate the beauty of nature. Ultimately, walking is a straightforward yet impactful type of exercise that can greatly influence both your physical and mental well-being. Adding regular walks to your daily routine can result in a healthier and more joyful life.

The Absence of PlayGrounds:

The absence of playgrounds in many communities is a concerning issue that has left youth with limited opportunities for physical activity and social interaction. Without designated spaces for play, children and teenagers may turn to video games as their primary form of entertainment. While video games can be a fun and engaging pastime, excessive screen time can negatively impact physical health and mental well-being. With playgrounds, youth can experience the benefits of outdoor play, such as developing gross motor skills, increasing physical fitness, and fostering social skills through peer interaction. Playgrounds provide children a safe and inclusive space to run, climb, and explore, promoting physical activity and creativity. When these spaces are not readily available, many youth may spend hours in front of a screen playing video games, which can harm their overall health and development. Communities should prioritize creating and maintaining playgrounds to ensure youth have access to play and physical activity opportunities. By providing safe and engaging spaces for children and teenagers to play, communities can help reduce the risk of sedentary lifestyles and promote healthy habits. Encouraging a balance between screen time and outdoor play can help prevent the negative impacts of video game addiction and support the overall well-being of youth.

Chapter Two

How Much Physical Activity Do You Need?

Here are the American Heart Association recommendations for adults.

Get at least 150 minutes per week of moderate-intensity aerobic activity or 75 minutes per week of vigorous aerobic activity (or a combination of both), preferably spread throughout the week.

Move More, Sit Less:

Get up and move throughout the day. Any activity is better than none. Even light-intensity activity can offset the serious health risks of being sedentary.

Add Intensity:

Moderate to vigorous aerobic exercise is best. Your heart will beat faster, and you'll breathe harder than normal. As you get used to being more active, increase your time and/or intensity to get more benefits.

Add Muscle:

Include moderate- to high-intensity muscle-strengthening activity (like resistance or weight training) at least twice a week.

Feel Better:

Physical activity is one of the best ways to keep your body and brain healthy.

It relieves stress, improves mood, gives you energy, helps with sleep and can lower your risk of chronic disease, including dementia and depression.Move more, with more intensity, and sit less.

https://www.heart.org/en/healthy-living/fitness/fitness-basics/aha-recs-for-physical-activity-infographic [3]

Before you start Jogging talk to your Doctor:

It can help you drop weight:

Walking, power-walking, jogging, and running — they all improve cardiovascular health and help prevent obesity. But one study, Trusted Source, found that if you want to boost your weight loss, you'll have more success if you pick up your pace.

The study doesn't distinguish between jogging and running. Instead, it focused on increased weight loss that occurred when participants ran instead of walked.

It can strengthen your immune system:

For the better part of a century, exercise scientists thought vigorous exercise could potentially leave you weakened and at risk for infection and disease. A closer look at the researchTrusted Source indicates the opposite is true.

Moderate exercise, like jogging, actually strengthens your body's response to illness. That holds true for both short-term illnesses, like upper respiratory tract infections, and long-term illnesses, like diabetes.

It has a positive effect on insulin resistance:

According to the Centers for Disease Control and Prevention (CDC)Trusted Source, more than 84 million Americans have prediabetes, a condition that can be reversed.

Insulin resistance is one of the markers of prediabetes. The cells in your body simply aren't responding to insulin, the hormone that keeps blood sugar levels in check.

The research found that regularly running or jogging decreased insulin resistance in study participants. Researchers noted that a decrease in body fat and inflammation might be behind the improvement in insulin resistance.

It can help you cope with depression:

Exercise has long been known to help people manage the symptoms of depression, but new science may help explain how. Elevated cortisol levels have been linked to depressive episodes. Cortisol is a hormone your body releases in response to stress. A 2018 study examined cortisol levels in people seeking treatment for depression. After 12 weeks of consistent exercise, those who exercised regularly throughout the study had reduced levels of cortisol throughout their entire day.Doctors at Mayo Clinic advise people who have symptoms of anxiety or depression to take up a physical activity they enjoy. Jogging is just one example. https://www.healthline.com/health/exercise-fitness/benefits-of-jogging#exercise-plateauThe American Heart Association Trusted Source recommends that you take good care of your feet before, during, and after jogging. Wear shoes made for running, talk to a pro about inserts or orthotics, and check for any blisters or swelling after you.

https://www.healthline.com/health/exercise-fitness/benefits-of-jogging#improve-depression. [4]

Endorphins and endocannabinoids:

Perhaps the most common neurotransmitters people think of in relation to exercise are endorphins. But lesser known neurotransmitters called endocannabinoids also play an important role in your brain when you're working out.

Endorphins block pain and increase sensations of pleasure, and exercise certainly increases your endorphin levels But recent research suggests that the euphoric feeling you get after a hard workout may result from endorphins and endocannabinoids working in tandem.

Endocannabinoids, in particular, are a group of neurotransmitters that are thought to be responsible for that "runner's high" — the feeling of calm euphoria that occurs after a strenuous workout.

https://www.healthline.com/health/depression/exercise#How-does-exercise-impact-the-brain? [5]

Dopamine:

Another impactful exercise-related neurotransmitter is dopamine.

Dopamine plays an important role in how you feel pleasure. It's also responsible for other processes in your body, such as regulating heart rate, sleep cycles, mood, attention, motivation, working memory, learning, and pain processing

Data is limited on which type of exercise best stimulates dopamine release, so more research is necessary.

Promotes neuroplasticity:

Neuroplasticity is the ability of your brain and nervous system to change their activity in response to internal or external stimuli .

This plays a huge role in learning new skills, activities, and languages.Some research suggests that exercise can promote neuroplasticity by increasing certain signaling factors

Increases oxygen supply to the brain:

As your heart starts to pump faster during exercise, it increases the oxygen supply to your brain.This results in certain changes to the blood vessels of your brain, promoting potential improvements in executive function, which includes working memory, flexible thinking, and self-control.In a 2021 study in 48 adults with mild cognitive impairment, researchers looked at the impact of exercise on blood flow to the cerebrum. This is the largest part of the brain and is responsible for higher intellectual function, sensory impulses, and motor activity They found that a 1-year moderate to vigorous exercise program increased cerebral blood flow and reduced the risk of further cognitive decline.

This suggests that regular physical activity can improve blood flow to important parts of your brain, in turn reducing your risk of conditions related to cognitive decline, such as Alzheimer's disease and stroke

According to science when you exercise, a number of neurotransmitters are released, including endorphins, endocannabinoids, and dopamine. Exercise also promotes neuroplasticity and increases oxygen supply to your brain.

Healthy eating and arthritis:

Your body works best when you eat a wide range of healthy foods. Most people find that they feel better if they eat a balanced and varied diet to get all the vitamins, minerals, antioxidants and other nutrients their body needs.

Try to eat a Mediterranean-style diet which includes fish, pulses, nuts, olive oil and plenty of fruit and vegetables. Eating a balanced diet and having an adequate fluid intake can also help provide you with better energy levels, help to maintain your weight, and give you a greater sense of wellbeing, which may improve your symptoms.

Always seek the advice of your doctor or dietitian before changing your diet. You may be restricting your food intake unnecessarily or taking too much of certain products (such as mineral supplements) that may have no impact on your condition at all. Some supplements may also interact with your medication.

https://www.betterhealth.vic.gov.au/health/conditionsandtreatments/arthritis-and-diet#arthritis-%E2%80%93-benefits-of-exercise. [6]

Calories burned in 30 minutes for people of three different weights.Calories burned chart by activity and weight, including walking, sports, and everyday household activities

While engaging in one of your favorite physical activities or exercises, you may have asked yourself, "How many calories do I burn while doing this?" Well, you may find your answer here. The table below lists the calories burned by doing dozens of activities listed by category (such as gym activities, training and sports activities, home repair etc.) for 30 minutes. Activities and exercises include walking (casual, race, and everything in between), swimming, jogging, yoga, and many more.

Calories Burned in 30-minute activities:

Gym Activities	125 Pound	155 Pound	188 Pound person
Weight Lifting:general	90	108	126
Aerobics:Water	120	1404	168
Stretching,Hatha Yoga	120	144	168
Calisthenics: moderate	135	162	189
Aerobics low impact	165	198	231
Stair Step Machine general	180	216	252
Weight Lifting:Vigorous	180	216	252
Aerobics.Step:how impact	210	252	294
Bicycling,Stationary Moderate	210	252	294
Rowing.Stationary moderate	210	252	294
Circuit Training :general	240	--	--
Rowing,Stationary Vigorous	255	369	440
Elliptical Trainer:general	270	324	378
Ski Machine:general	285	342	399
Aerobics,Step:high Impact	300	630	420
Bicycling,Stationary Vigorous:	315	278	441

https://www.health.harvard.edu/diet-and-weight-loss/calories-burned-in-30-minutes-for-people-of-three-different-weights. [7]

Regular exercise reduces arthritis symptoms:

What causes rheumatoid arthritis?

We don't know what causes the immune system to malfunction and attack the joints, but it appears that your genes may play a role. Other factors such as hormones, infection (by an unknown bacteria or virus), emotional distress or environmental triggers (such as cigarette smoke or pollutants) may be involved.

What are the symptoms of rheumatoid arthritis?

The most common symptoms of rheumatoid arthritis include:

- swelling, pain and heat in the joints, usually starting in the smaller joints of the hands or feet
- stiffness in the joints, especially in the morning
- persistent mental and physical tiredness (fatigue)
- the same joints on both sides of the body being affected

Less common symptoms may include weight loss, inflammation of other body parts (such as the lungs or eyes) or rheumatoid nodules (fleshy lumps below the elbows or on hands or feet).

Rheumatoid arthritis can occur at any age, but usually appears between the ages of 30 and 60. It affects women more often than men.

The course and severity of rheumatoid arthritis varies from person to person. Symptoms may change from day to day.

At times your symptoms (such as pain, fatigue and inflammation) may become more intense. This is a flare, or flare-up. Flares are unpredictable and can seem to come out of nowhere.

https://www.betterhealth.vic.gov.au/heal [8]th/conditionsandtreatments/rheumatoid-arthritis#your-joints-and-rheumatoid-arthritis

Arthritis – benefits of exercise:

Arthritis can cause pain, stiffness and often inflammation in one or more joints or muscles. Regular exercise can reduce some of the symptoms of arthritis, and improve your joint mobility and strength.Regular exercise has many health benefits for people with arthritis. Exercise can:

- Aid joint lubrication and nourishment
- ease your joint pain and stiffness
- improve flexibility

- build muscular strength
- improve your balance
- help you sleep better
- improve posture
- improve or maintain the density of your bones
- improve overall health and fitness
- lower stress levels
- Improve your mood
- Help you maintain a healthy body weight.

https://www.betterhealth.vic.gov.au/health/conditionsandtreatments/arthritis-and-exercise#arthritis-%E2%80%93-benefits-of-exercise

In conclusion, It is essential to prioritize your health and consult with healthcare professionals regarding any health concerns or conditions you may have. They will be able to provide you with the necessary guidance to ensure that your exercise and dietary plans are safe and suitable for your specific needs.

References

- Sahih al-Bukhari 5199 [183] [1]-
- Sahih al-Bukhari 6412 [2]
- www.heart.org/en/healthy-living/fitness/fitness-basics/aha-recs-for-physical-activity-infographic [3]
- https://www.healthline.com/health/exercise-fitness/benefits-of-jogging#improve-depression. [4]
- https://www.healthline.com/health/depression/exercise#How-does-exercise-impact-the-brain? [5]
- https://www.betterhealth.vic.gov.au/health/conditionsandtreatments/arthritis-and-diet#arthritis-%E2%80%93-benefits-of-exercise. [6]
- https://www.health.harvard.edu/diet-and-weight-loss/calories-burned-in-30-minutes-for-people-of-three-different-weights. [7]
- https://www.betterhealth.vic.gov.au/heal [8]

www.ingramcontent.com/pod-product-compliance
Lightning Source LLC
LaVergne TN
LVHW041003150826
845672LV00002B/846

* 9 7 9 8 8 9 4 7 5 2 9 3 8 *